Paleo Diet for Weight Loss and Wellness

Get Slim and Fit the Easy Way

Matthew Noll

© 2016

TABLE OF CONTENTS

INTRODUCTION

You are reading this Paleo diet book means that somewhere in your mind you have decided that you want a healthier body and a better life. This is one of the greatest things you have ever done for your life. You can never take your body for granted and it is nice that you have finally decided to work on it. **Paleo Diet for Weight Loss and Wellness: Get Slim and Fit the Easy Way** is an all-embracing book on Paleo eating. You will find everything related to the topic in this book. The best part is that the book does not contain any links or hidden references to any kind of information.

With a gliding flow of information, you will learn about Paleo eating in this book. In the concluding chapters, you will also get enlightened about beginning this diet if you have any confusion regarding the same. Since Paleo diet belongs to the Stone Age, you might face some difficulties in the beginning phase and your body might not adapt it completely. You need to overcome this time and emerge victorious.

You will start observing the visible results even if others around you do not. Your body feels energized when you are on a healthy diet. You tend to face the challenges of daily life in a better way and deal with stress much more easily. Among so many benefits of Paleo diet, the biggest one is that you lose weight significantly and your body gets leaner. Everybody around you compliments you and that is the greatest motivation.

Your friends and family will want to know the secret behind your makeover. Feel free to share the tips and be the master of a healthy body. If you successfully deal with the challenges of Paleo transition in the first few weeks, you can do it easily for the rest of your life. If you get bored with Paleo eating after a long time, you can take a break and bring some non-Paleo foods for a while. Nevertheless, these breaks should not be permanent because just one bar of chocolate can ruin weeks of your efforts, and you would certainly not want that.

Just go ahead reading this book and have a great time eating as much as you want with Paleo!

CHAPTER 1

What is Paleo Diet?

The Paleo diet is an extremely healthy way you can adopt right now. With our modern lifestyle, we have forgotten our genetic needs for food and have started eating unnecessary junk. Paleo diet is not a new revolution of food, but it belongs to the Stone Age. Paleo regime works in conjunction with your genetics in order to help you become strong, energetic, lean, and never fat.

There have been numerous researches in Dermatology Biology, Ophthalmology, Biochemistry, and many other branches of science and medicine, which prove that our modern diet is full of refined foods, sugar, and trans-fat. This diet is the root cause of harmful degenerative ailments such as cancer, obesity, heart disease, diabetes, Parkinson's, depression, Alzheimer's, and infertility.

The staple components of Paleo diet are eggs, fish, and meat. Even though different experts have varied opinions about this diet, a few experts say that Paleo eaters should rely on lean meat for better results, and the majority of them believe that one should eat organic meat. Organic meat is the one that comes from animals that ate natural foods while they lived.

Although this diet encourages non-starchy vegetables, but not legumes and beans are not supported. This also implies you can eat spinach and kale, but not carrots and potatoes. Some of the fruits are also classified as Paleo foods. For receiving protein and fat from sources, excluding fish and meat, from sources like nuts, coconut oil, olive oil in limited quantities. The list of forbidden foods majorly includes starches and sugars. Since you cannot eat grains, you have to avoid bread. You cannot consume dairy products, but you can eat dairy substitutes like almond or coconut milk. Even if meat is encouraged in Paleo diet, one should not eat processed meat like sausage and bacon.

You might have heard good and bad things about Paleo diet. Some of these things are actually true and many of the negative comments are just myths. They are circulated because of the fact that Paleo diet demands a little strictness in regime and not many people can follow it. You have to be much disciplined with your diet and incorporate into your lifestyle. When some people cannot do it, they give rise to negative myths about this diet and hence scare people away from this awesome diet plan.

Paleo diet is designed to give you a lean, yet strong body. Once you adopt it completely and start loving it, you will never want to get back to your old foods. Even if you eat food from your old regime, neither will you like it, nor your body will accept it.

Is Paleo diet helpful for diabetics?

Yes, definitely, Paleo diet does work well for diabetes type 2. However, as stated above, you must consult your doctor if you have diabetes. The Paleo diet can reverse the symptoms of Type-2 diabetes, which is insulin resistant. Compared to Mediterranean diet, Paleo diet can combat diabetes in more effective manner.

Think about a time when you are allowed to have ice cream with all the meals you have. Even if you are a passionate lover of ice cream, you would start avoiding it in a few weeks. Then, after a few months, if you are forced to eat it just for the sake of friendship, you may eventually start hating it. A time would come when you will reject a bowl of your favorite ice cream. This is true in case of your body as well. If you feed your body with sugary, cheap foods that are most common in an American diet, your body will desensitize itself from such foods just because it does not need or want them.

Our body needs a certain amount of energy; when your body

reaches that verge, the cells of the body reject the food and amass it as fat. In case you do not control your sugar intake for a long time, your body becomes sensitive of insulin, which implies your body would not identify the sugar whether your cells are saturated or not.

If you consume Paleo diet even for short term, it improves your glucose tolerance and blood pressure levels. Insulin secretion is decreased and lipid profiles are improved.

Cardio Vascular Disease

Cardio vascular disease is the topmost cause of deaths in America. Our modern studies show that the hunter- gatherers virtually never suffered any stroke or heart attack. Since the food that Paleo diet recommends provides you the nutrients you need from all natural sources, you do not have to worry about most diseases. However, you cannot guarantee that you will never suffer from any disease because other factors from our modern lifestyle are also responsible for many diseases. As a matter of fact, you can significantly bring down their probability.

Autoimmunity

Autoimmunity is referred to a process which makes our own

immune system damage our body. Typically, the immune system is meant to defend us from parasitic, bacterial, and viral infections. It recognizes a foreign organism and attacks it to clear any infection. For example, when a person undergoes organ transplant, sometimes the body does not accept it and rejects its tissues. Even if the tissues are matched beforehand, the body does not accept the new organs.

A similar procedure takes place in autoimmunity when our own tissues are confused for foreign invaders and the immune system starts invading it. Some examples of autoimmunity are Multiple Sclerosis, Lupus, Rheumatoid Arthritis, and Vitiligo, etc. Autoimmunity plays a major role in some of the seemingly unrelated conditions like infertility, Schizophrenia, and several types of cancer.

The important factor to note here is that these apparently unrelated diseases have a common ground: damage to intestinal lining. It occurs when undigested large particles of food enter the inner parts of our body, which is known as autoimmune response and leaky gut. There are several examples of patients who were able to reverse the symptoms of leaky gut and Multiple Sclerosis just by adopting Paleo diet.

CHAPTER 2

What you Gain from Paleo Diet

For most of the health conscious people, the only assurance is enough that Paleo delivers great results. Improvement in blood lipids, lower sting from autoimmunity, and weight loss is good enough as proof. However, there are many people who are not contended with blind recommendations of this diet, even if they are about exercise and nutrition. They want to know the reason behind every single recommendation, and this is not wrong, in fact. We all have the right to know what we are eating and why we are eating. The good news is that Paleo diet has stood the test of time and has a reason for every good word it says.

With a simple shift in foods, this diet aims to remove the cuisines that are not good for our health, and add those which increase the intake of minerals, vitamins, and antioxidants. Paleolithic diet is new for the majority of people and of course, many questions are raised. If you are also new to this diet, you must educate yourself about this diet and get into the depth of it. Let us go through some of the tremendous benefits of Paleo diet.

Balanced levels of blood glucose

Since you avoid refined sugar in Paleo diet, it becomes easier to prevent soaring of blood sugar in your body. When you experience sugar crash in the body, you are able to avoid sensation of fatigue. However, if you are a diabetic, you must consult your doctor before you jump into a new routine. On the other hand, if you want to avoid diabetes, you can straightaway start this diet. And in any case, Paleo diet is good to lose weight, watch the blood sugar level.

Leaner muscles

Since you will be eating a lot of meat in Paleo diet, you can be sure of getting plenty protein from your food. Your muscles will be well fed with the amount of protein you eat, and this is particularly helpful if you are engaged in weightlifting. You can recall the physiques of men from Stone Age; they were never shown with heavy bodies in their stone carvings, which are the true representation of their society. Those people never had excess fat around their tummy or thighs, and they had well developed muscles. People of that age were lean and strong, who were capable of fighting carnivorous animals with bare hands.

Although nobody expects you to become a person of that sort, but you can definitely gain some muscle from this diet for handle the challenges of your life in a better way.

Avoid gluten and wheat

When you cut down on grains, such as wheat, you can automatically get rid of gluten, which means that you are following the gluten free diet simultaneously. You must have read earlier that gluten is not good for our digestive system and it makes us gain weight. Even if you do not have gluten sensitivity or Celiac disease, you can have an improved body makeup by cutting down on gluten.

Makes you feel full for a long time

If you start some other food regime, you might feel that you are constantly hungry throughout the day. However, with Paleo diet, you eat more meat, i.e. healthy fat and protein, which keeps your stomach full for a long time and avoids food cravings. It means that you do not have to eat more fat or carbohydrates again and again. You will not feel like cheating on your diet since you do not feel hungry more often. If you consume the right amount of proteins and fats from meat and carbohydrates and fiber from fruits and vegetables, you will not even feel hungry between the meals.

No need of counting calories

If you have gone through a diet plan that makes you count your carbohydrates and calories, you must know how painful it is to do that. The Paleo diet is essentially easy and simple to follow. There are hardly any limitations and rules about how much food you need to have every day. This makes it fun and simple to stick to your plan every time you eat. You do not have to check yourself and that makes your plan successful. You just need to eat without complicating your meals; just the way our ancestors ate.

Prevents diseases

Paleo diet includes majorly anti-inflammatory foods; it cuts down on foods that cause inflammation. Moreover, Paleo foods contain phytonutrients and antioxidants, which are obviously known to fight cancer and prevent heart ailments. Junk and fast food are known to cause maximum illnesses and diseases. Therefore, when you limit yourself from these foods, you can be sure of well-being and healing your body.

Better sleep

When you cut down on additives and chemicals in standard sources of food, you will observe that the body gets naturally tired at night, because of a chemical called serotonin. This chemical is released by your brain when it is the ideal time to have sleep and your body is not burdened by other chemicals of junk food. When you begin feeling sleepy, it is best that you sleep in more or less 30 minutes. You might observe that you start feeling tired earlier than before at night, and you feel more energized in the morning. It means that your body is getting to terms with circadian rhythm.

Keep away from processed Foods

In the last century, many harmful chemicals have entered our foods. You will be surprised to know that many foods are not allowed in Paleo diet as a result of processing involved. More than 90% of the world population is habitual of eating these foods. You may feel difficulty in shunning packed foods and dairy products. You may have to face some time of psychological and physical adjustment and criticism from your friends and family towards a better way of lifestyle. Then, you will notice how deeply you have set in your modern conveniences.

Keep away from fast food

Fast food not just makes you fat, but also deteriorates your health, and this is nothing new to us. Even if we know that this food is playing havoc with our health, still we have a real hard time giving them up. Just keep one thing in mind that your ancestors enjoyed much better health than you and they never depended on McDonalds. The fast food chains keep your health as their last priority and their profits as first. Paleo gives you a break from this vicious circle.

Cuts out calories and carbohydrates

You need to cut out on soft drinks, energy drinks, packed juices, and many other beverages that are loaded with sugar and chemicals. The reason is simple- they are processed drinks and hence, you need to stay away from them. You can, although, have a few herbal teas. It will definitely make you feel better, help you lose weight, and have better levels of sustained energy round the clock. With Paleo diet, every calorie and carbohydrate you take is meant to serve your body for better.

More energy

If the Paleo foods are combined in the right amount, you get a balanced meal that consists of carbohydrates, fats, proteins and other minerals in just right proportion. Moreover, you are taking all the nutrients from natural sources. You do not have to depend on energy drinks, or caffeinated beverages to gain energy. Moreover, you never fall short of calories in Paleo diet, unlike other diets. You can eat whenever you want, without feeling guilty. You are never out of energy when you need it. You have your fuel, i.e. food at your disposal all the time.

Detoxification effects

In Paleo diet, you bring down the consumption of a lot of products that exterminate your body, such as trans-fats, caffeine, MSG, gluten, refined sugar, and many more. By cutting down on these things, you are giving a healthy break to your body. The Paleo fruits give you more antioxidants and the vegetables give you more phytonutrients and fiber. Your body is, thus, purged from the waste that builds up inside. The detoxifying effect is provided to your body, which is actually proven with many Paleo eaters. They have stated that they feel clear headed and lighter after they adopted Paleo diet. The best part about Paleo is that you do not have to take your body to extreme levels of fasting. Therefore, Paleo eating is a kind of lazy detoxification.

Keeps matters simple

Following many forms of other diets may make you mentally tired. Practically, no human being can constantly think of what they should eat, when they should eat, and what is good for health, etc. Paleo keeps matters really simple so that your mind is not occupied with food all the time. You will be amazed to find out the freedom you get from constant thinking. You can obviously use this free time for more important things.

Increases the consumption of fruits and vegetables

Most Americans cannot meet their daily requirement of fruits and vegetables, just because they are stuffed with junk food all the time. Paleo present these *healthy* and *obligatory* foods in a better way so that you do not feel burdened to eat them. Rather, you will feel motivated to consume them. The main aim of Paleo diet is to keep your tongue satiated along with your stomach so that you do not feel tempted to eat fast food or junk food.

Helps you lose weight effortlessly

With Paleo regime, your weight naturally comes down while you eat more fat! Doesn't it sound amazing? Yes, it is true. Since your body is consuming healthy fats, it adapts to using bad fats for energy. The interesting phenomenon about Paleo diet is that the more you enjoy this regime, the more weight you lose. On the other hand, if you resent your plan, or crave for things that you cannot eat, you are bound to fail on this regime and may sacrifice your health.

Circle of life

Eating meat in Paleo diet does not mean that you are placing a burden on environment because you are eating pasture- raised eggs and meat. It implies that the meat comes from animals that have lived their full lives. Typically, chickens and cows roam around the pasture in conjunction as this forms synergy. In a farm, chickens roam around the cows and eat the bugs and larvae found lying under cow pies. The cow pie gets broken into smaller forms to fertilize the grass. This grass ultimately supplies food for cow. This beautiful process is the circle of life.

This diet is of course natural for animals and it also gives the humans a long catalog of nutrients, while they are eaten as meat. Moreover, eggs that come from pastured hens contain 10 times more of omega-3 compared to eggs that come from hens reared in factories.

Less allergies

Paleo diet recommends that you must minimize the consumption of food that is supposed to cause allergies. Some people cannot digest dairy products and grains. Paleo diet is criticized sometimes because it does not allow even whole grains. However, the fact is that grains are not completely avoided. You can eat oats more frequently.

CHAPTER 3

What you lose with Paleo Diet

While having a long list of advantages, there are only a few disadvantages of Paleo diet. The only good word that can be said here is that, choose the best and leave the rest. Still, you must be aware of the downsides of Paleo, even if they are minimal.

Lack of a few vitamins

Some of the potentially beneficial nutrients such as calcium and vitamin D that are found in abundance in dairy products are not sufficiently found in Paleo foods. These vitamins are found to prevent diseases akin to fractures, osteoporosis and many other bone issues.

Essential proteins are not provided

Meat is eaten only thrice a week in Paleo diet, and many other beans and legumes are not recommended for nutrition. Therefore, some people may be deprived of some essential nutrients, which may result in weakness, tendency to develop some infections, and loss of mass in muscles.

More amount of salt

Most foods of Paleo diet include significant amount of salt, which is not recommended in many other diet plans. Although a moderate amount of salt is needed to maintain metabolic rate in body and to moderate functioning of thyroid. However, if salt is consumed in higher doses, it may lead to high blood pressure and cardiac diseases.

Over and under cooking

Whether it is over cooking or under cooking, it destroys the essential nutrients of food and affects the attributes of calories that we consume. Under cooked vegetables are found to result in parasitic infestation for Paleo eaters, which may lead to several chronic health problems.

How safe is Paleo diet?

We have to take the criticisms of Paleo diet a bit seriously since we cannot take for granted that our ancestors used to eat meat all the time. Different cavemen had different surroundings and that made changes to their diet as well. When they lived in proximity to sea, their diet included more of sea food, and if they lived close to jungles, they ate more of animal meat. And in any case, they ate a lot of fruits and vegetables. That is why; we cannot safely say that consuming a

19

lot of protein is good for health.

Is Paleo diet really healthy?

Even after consuming several healthy foods, the Paleo diet remains deficient in vitamin D and calcium. Therefore, it makes Paleo diet extremely potentially healthy, but some people may need more of these nutrients, which may make them partially deficient. Simultaneously, protein and saturated fat is consumed in abundance in Paleo diet, which raises the chances of heart diseases, kidney ailments, and many cancers.

You might have heard that we should reduce dairy and carbohydrates in our foods. However, our body needs complex carbohydrates, which can be had from oats, fruits, and vegetables. They work as an important fuel for muscle and brain activity. We must consume refined carbohydrates that add needless calories and ingredients, but a little amount of protein and fiber.

Consuming dairy products is subjective matter, more related to choice of a person. In spite of this, you must not limit its consumption to the extremes. Even if you do, you must replace dairy foods with alternative sources of food that can provide you vitamin D and calcium. Advocates of Paleo diet often say that dairy encourages inflammation, but there have been some researches, which show that low fat products of dairy are capable of decreasing inflammation in blood.

For some people, Paleo may not work for lasting weight loss, since it becomes difficult to be dedicated to a diet that places several restrictions in terms of food categories. Concerning overall health, this diet may give rise to lipids such as low-density lipoprotein or LDL; it increases the chances of heart ailments. If your body does not receive enough calcium, you may develop symptoms of rickets, bone fractures, and osteoporosis. Moreover, extremely low intake of calcium may result in overuse of fats in the body for energy; the process called ketosis. You must consult your doctor if you plan to stay on Paleo diet for long time, especially if you have kidney, pancreatic, or heart disease. You must also consult the physician if you wish to stay on the low carbohydrate kind of Paleo diet.

Should you adopt Paleo diet?

As a beginning milestone towards a healthy diet, you can adopt Paleo diet. Nevertheless, once you achieve your fitness goals, you must add lentils, whole grains, nuts, beans, and nonfat or low fat dairy sources, or other sources of calcium like tofu, dark leafy greens, and almond or soymilk. You must choose your sources of protein carefully, and lay emphasis on quality than quantity.

CHAPTER 4

List of Paleo and non-Paleo foods

The list of Paleo foods, which you can comfortably eat, is as follows: *Grass-fed meats, Seeds, Fresh fruits, Fish/seafood, Eggs, Fresh vegetables, Nuts, Healthy oils such as olive, walnut, macadamia, flaxseed, avocado, coconut.*

Avoid eating *Cereal grains, Dairy, Legumes like peanuts, refined sugar, processed foods, Potatoes, extremely salty foods, Junk/Candy/ processed food, and Refined* vegetable oils.

Meats in Paleo Diet

You can eat any kind of meat in Paleo, but stay away from processed meats and high- fat meats.

Poultry, Chicken breast, Turkey, Pork tenderloin, Turkey, Steak, Turkey, Veal, Bacon, Ground beef, Pork, Grass-fed beef, Chicken leg, Chicken thigh, Lamb rack, Chicken wings, Shrimp, Clams, Lobster, Salmon, Buffalo, Venison steaks, New York steak, Bison rib eye, Lamb chops, Bison, Rabbit, Bison steaks, Goat, Elk, Bison jerky, Emu, Goose, Bison sirloin,

Kangaroo, Bear, Beef jerky, Eggs (chicken, duck, or goose), Reindeer, Wild boar, Turtle, Pheasant, Ostrich, Quail, Chuck steak, Lean veal, and Rattlesnake.

Fish in Paleo Diet

Bass, Salmon, Mackerel, Sardines, Halibut, Tuna, Shark, Red snapper, Sunfish, Tilapia, Swordfish, Trout, Walleye

Seafood in Paleo Diet

Crab, Crayfish, Crawfish, Shrimp, Lobster, Clams, Scallops, Oysters

Vegetables in Paleo Diet

Asparagus, Artichoke hearts, Avocado, Brussels sprouts, Spinach, Carrots, Celery, Zucchini, Broccoli, Cabbage, Cauliflower, Peppers Parsley, Green onions, and Eggplant

Starchy vegetables

Since these vegetables are starchy, they should be eaten in moderation, particularly for those trying to shed weight. Acorn squash, Butternut squash, Yam, Beets, Sweet potato, Paleo Diet Fats/ Oils

Paleo oils

Olive oil, Coconut oil, Macadamia oil, Grass-fed butter, Avocado oil.

Nuts in Paleo diet

Cashews, Almonds, Hazelnuts, Pine nuts, Pecans, Pumpkin seeds, Macadamia nuts, Sunflower seeds, Walnuts.

Since peanuts are nuts, but legumes, they should not be eaten.

Fruits in Paleo Diet

If you want to lose weight with Paleo diet, you must watch your fruit intake since they contain fructose. You can still have 2-3 servings of fruits every day.

Apple, Blackberries, Avocado, Papaya, Plums, Peaches, Mango, Blueberries, Lychee, Grapes, Strawberries, Lemon, Watermelon, guava, Lime, Pineapple, Raspberries, Tangerine, Cantaloupe, Figs, Bananas, Oranges

Non- Paleo foods that you must avoid

It might be difficult to quit these foods completely, but if you do, the effort is worth it.

Dairy, Cheese, Butter, Cottage cheese, Skim milk, Non-fat dairy creamer, 2% milk, Dairy spreads, Whole milk, Cream cheese, Yogurt, powdered milk, Pudding, Ice milk, Frozen yogurt, Low fat milk, Soft drinks, Ice cream.

Coke and other sweetened beverages are packed with high amounts of sugar and hence, they must be avoided. Mountain Dew, Coke, Pepsi, Sprite, etc

Fruit Juices

Mango juice, Orange juice, Apple juice, Grape juice, Chinola juice, Strawberry juice, Starfruit juice

Grains

Anything that contains grains must be completely avoided.

Cereals, English muffins, Bread, Toast, Triscuits, Sandwiches, Wheat Thins, Oatmeal, Crackers, Cream of wheat, Corn syrup, Corn, Wheat, corn syrup (High-fructose), Pancakes, Beer, Hash browns, Pasta, Lasagna, Fettuccini, Legumes

Legumes

Black beans, Fava beans, Broad beans, Garbanzo beans, Kidney beans, Horse beans, Lima beans, Adzuki beans, Mung beans, Navy beans, Red beans, Pinto beans, Green beans, White beans, String beans, Peas, Chickpeas, Black-eyed peas, Snow peas, Peanuts, Sugar snap peas, Peanut butter, Lentils, Lupines, Soybeans, Tofu, Mesquite, and other beans.

Artificial Sweeteners

Avoid all artificial sweeteners. If you want to sweeten your food or drinks, you can use honey, stevia, or maple syrup.

Fatty Meats

All kinds of fat meat should be strictly avoided. Spam, low-quality meats, Hot dogs

Salty Foods

Ketchup, French fries

Snacks

Pretzels, Chips, Triscuits, Wheat Thins, Cookies, Sun Chips, Pastries, Starchy Vegetables

Starchy vegetables

Sweet potatoes, Potatoes, Yucca, Butternut squash, Batata,

Acorn squash, Beets, Yam

Energy Drinks

Red Bull, 5-Hour Energy, Rockstar, Monster, Starbucks Refreshers, Vault, Mountain Dew MDX, XS Energy Drink

Alcohol

No kinds of alcohol are allowed in Paleo diet. Beer, Tequila, Whiskey, Rum, Alcohol, Vodka, and mixers

Sweets

Candy bars, Snickers Peanut Butter, Snickers, 100 Grand, Milky Way, Butterfinger, Reese's, M&Ms, Payday, Skittles, Twizzlers, Red Vines, Hershey's, Almond Joy, Nestle Crunch, Mounds, Reese's Pieces, Reese's Fast Break, Peanut Twix.

CHAPTER 5

How to Start Paleo Eating

The most difficult step in beginning a journey is the first step. However, you can always gather courage and start eating Paleo.

1. Makeover your kitchen

You might think that you have mounds of willpower and you can avoid any temptations of eating non- Paleo food, but the truth is that if you keep anything that is not allowed in Paleo, you will eat it someday. That is why; you need to do away with anything that you cannot eat, including raw material. Since unhealthy foods are easily available, they tempt much more than healthy foods.

The best way is to keep all healthy things around you, so that even if you are terribly hungry, you will get your hands on Paleo foods. Roughly, you will want to throw everything that comes in a packet, jar, or can. If something contains more than 3-4 ingredients, discard it. If you doubt something, discard it.

Do not think that you are wasting food; you are discarding

disease-causing elements from your house. You may want to donate it to someone who will happily accept it.

2. Go shopping

Now when you have emptied most of you kitchen and refrigerator, you need to refill them with healthy things. You can read the Paleo foods list given below and buy whatever you require for a week. Some of these things can be bought for a long time.

Since most Paleo foods will not contain more than two ingredients, you will not have to read many labels. That will also save you a lot of headache that you used to have earlier counting calories.

3. Learn cooking

You will have to mix and cook some Paleo ingredients to cook a healthy meal for yourself. Therefore, whatsoever about cooking terrifies you, overcome your fears and learn cooking. You will thank yourself that you did. You will definitely enjoy it as well, once you start receiving the benefits.

Do not indulge yourself in cooking elaborate cuisines at first. Start with easy things and then you can jump to complicated dishes.

4. Exercise

You simply need to be active when you are eating a lot of fat. Recall that the cave dwellers used to be extremely active when it came to their daily lives. That is why; they were able to digest the heavy meat of animals and sea creatures, and still remain fit. Similarly, you need to exercise at least for a while daily, if you are eating Paleo foods. You can join sports with your friends or just go for jogging alone. The broad idea is to get started with at least something.

5. Sleep

You will need plenty of sleep, and that counts to brownie points of Paleo diet for most of us. To achieve perfect wellness and health, you need to sleep well to perform well in athletics, improve your mood, increase energy, boost your immune system, enhance your memory, increase mental focus, tolerate stress, and decrease the risk of heart disease, Type 2 diabetes, and obesity.

You can use these tips to have a good sleep:

Turn off the television and computer

Fix a time to watch TV and just turn it off after that. The electronic gadgets tend to interfere with our sleep. Do not get tempted by the TV shows or movies you miss. After a few days, your improved health will show you the benefits of not watching TV. If you cannot sleep without TV, you can prefer reading a book.

Bring blinds or dark curtains

If the light from streets or from some other room interferes with your sleep, you can pull the blinds or dark curtains.

Make your room cooler

When our body is too warm, it cannot indulge into deep sleep. That is why; we tend to get addicted to air conditioners. Try to cool your room naturally if the weather in your region allows. Bring the temperature of your room to a comfortable temperature to sleep better and longer.

Make your sleeping time consistent

Try to sleep and wake up at a consistent time. It will make

your body healthier.

6. Watch out for these things

You may face difficulties in adjusting to your new eating habits, since your body is undergoing the process of cleansing, releasing toxins, switching to a fat burning machine, and getting into a healthier state. Nevertheless, you do not have to get discouraged and keep up your enthusiasm for the first few weeks. Some of your friends and family members might even discourage you, but you just have to keep in mind that you are changing for better.

Tell your friends and family about your eating preferences

Everybody who remains around you or eats with you should know about your eating habits so that they do not force you to eat non-Paleo foods. They might even get defensive since they are eating everything that you are flatly refusing, but do not get discouraged and politely refuse.

Let your results talk

You do not have to brag about your new food habits once you start your Paleo regime. Just go ahead with it for a few weeks and let the results show. You will see people asking you the secret of high energy and a lean body very soon.

Keep learning

Never stop learning about Paleo lifestyle. You can Google about it often and read books about it. When you have plenty information, you are less likely to commit mistakes. Moreover, you can educate others in the right perspective about Paleo.

CONCLUSION

After reading so much about Paleo, doesn't it feel good to start your journey? It gives certain motivation to begin a new lifestyle that can give you so much in terms of good health, enhanced energy and metabolism and a great body. Having a beautiful body indeed feels good and you feel even better when you receive compliments.

We live in a cruel world and we have to be physically and mentally fit to face the challenges. This same cruel world takes a beautiful form when you have the energy to absorb the shocks. If you are weak and frail, or even overweight, you will never feel like putting in efforts face up to the tests of your personal and professional life.

Since you have gone through the basics of Paleo diet, you can do yourself one big favor- learn cooking. Sticking to Paleo diet will become significantly easy if you learn cooking. You will definitely enjoy more when you know how to feed yourself since you cannot order Paleo food every time; neither have you had the option to do so every time.

You can buy a Paleo cuisines book to learn Paleo cooking. Start with easy recipes to get the hang of basic cooking and then you can proceed to dishes that are more complicated. Do not stop experimenting and eat a variety of foods at work or at home. You must have read the tips to start Paleo eating, but reading is no use if you do not implement it right away. If you let a few weeks pass before you start, you might never do it. Just get up and make a to-do list to get started.

Good luck for you new journey with Paleo eating!

www.ingramcontent.com/pod-product-compliance
Lightning Source LLC
Chambersburg PA
CBHW030547290526
45786CB00004B/1910